ELEVATE YOUR
energy

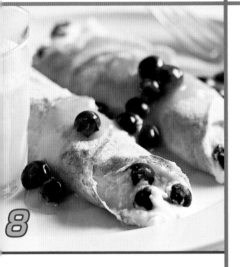

8

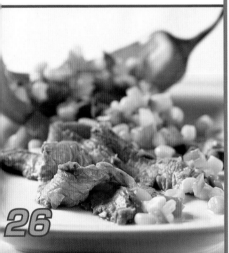

26

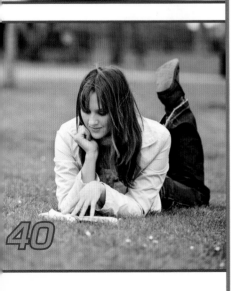

40

recipes

start the day right	8
go meatless	18
power meals	26
the lighter side	34
healthy sides	44

energize

empty on energy?	2
z's count!	14
the new power lunch	24
beat the afternoon slump	33
life in the slow lane	40
healthy snacks	48

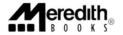

Des Moines, Iowa

Copyright © 2008 Meredith Corporation
First Edition. Printed in China.
Excerpted from *Boost Your Energy*, 2006.
ISBN: 978-0-696-24088-1

empty on energy?

by Donna Shields, M.S., R.D.

Life's complicated and hectic pace can physically and emotionally drain a person, even when things go smoothly. Add into the mix a life-changing event, such as a family death, a career change, or a move, and you've got the makings for a total energy meltdown. Even so, many small steps can help lighten the load and restore your energy levels so you can better handle what life dishes out.

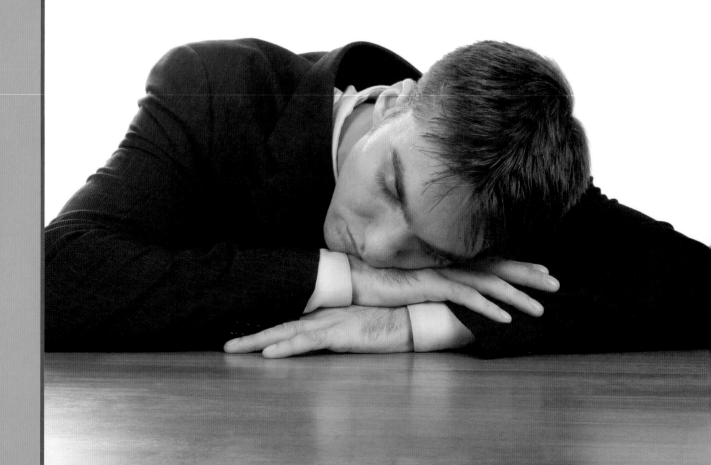

Small Steps to Refuel Yourself

Many different factors sap energy levels, and most can be fixed with just a little tweaking. A simple change in routine or a discussion with a health-care provider or counselor may be all you need. In any case, here's a good overview for assessing what may be causing your personal energy drain.

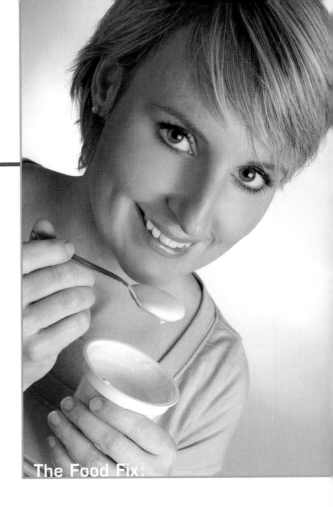

The Food Fix:

Photographs: www.istockphoto.com/Alex Gumerov (opposite), Dušan Zidar (upper right)

Not Getting Enough Sleep?

Getting enough sleep sounds so simple, but most people are walking around sleep-deprived, and it shows in their attitudes and energy levels. Lack of sleep causes headaches, an inability to focus, and impaired judgment. Sleep apnea, which causes unconscious awakening many times during the night, leaves you feeling completely tired in the morning and requires medical attention.

The Fix: While some people squeak by with just five hours of sleep per night, most folks require a solid eight hours. Make your bedroom a soothing and inviting place. New pillowcases or a comforter could do the trick. Opt for soft lamp lighting in place of a bright ceiling fixture. Do not drink anything several hours before bedtime so your sleep isn't interrupted by a bathroom trip. Sleep is enhanced by a brain chemical called serotonin, which is produced from the amino acid tryptophan and gives a person a soothing, relaxing feeling. A small bedtime snack of protein and carbohydrate, such as yogurt, cheese, or whole grain or graham crackers, enhances serotonin production and helps you drift off more easily.

Are You Stressed?

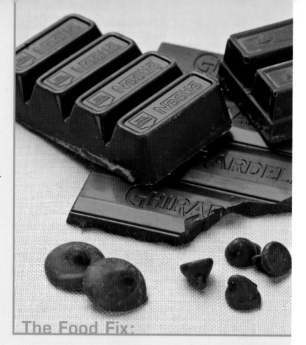

Stress, which takes its toll physically and mentally, comes at us from many different directions; financial worries, poor relationships with a partner or children, job concerns, and just not enough time to accomplish our priorities all add stress to our lives.

The Fix: While you may not be able to change a situation, how you approach it makes all the difference. Many women find that bonding with other women provides needed emotional support during stressful times.

The Food Fix:

Grabbing a comfort food, especially if it's chocolate, may not be such a bad idea. Dark chocolate, just like chile peppers, helps stimulate endorphins, brain chemicals that help relieve stress and pain.

Not Enough Exercise?

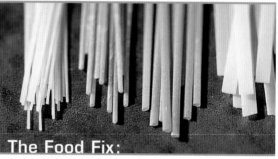

When you feel sluggish and run-down, the last thing you want to do is exercise. The less you move, the less you want to do, and the snowball effect of inactivity goes into motion.

The Fix: Aerobic exercise actually boosts energy levels, and the exercise session doesn't need to be long or strenuous. A 15-minute walk on your lunch break or raking leaves in the front yard for a half hour on a Saturday could give you the exercise you need.

The Food Fix:

Exercise requires fuel, and the body's preferred source of fuel is carbohydrates, especially the complex type. Brown rice side dishes, multigrain pastas, and 100-percent whole wheat bread add fiber to your diet and provide a slow, steady release of energy to your body as opposed to the spike-and-crash results of a highly refined sugar diet. Before you grab an energy bar, check to see if sugar ranks high on the ingredients list.

Too Many Medications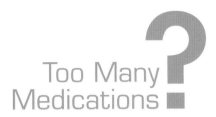

Prescription and over-the-counter drugs drag down energy levels. This can be especially true if you take multiple medications that cause drug interactions.

The Fix: If you suspect drug interactions are a problem, take all of your medications to your health-care provider for a thorough assessment. Don't overlook vitamin, herbal, and dietary supplements, as they factor into the equation, too.

The Food Fix: Vitamins, minerals, and antioxidants all play an important role in the body's ability to keep going full steam ahead, and magnesium seems to be particularly important in sustaining energy. A study conducted by the U.S. Department of Agriculture's Human Nutrition Research Center, Grand Forks, North Dakota, shows that postmenopausal women with low magnesium levels need more energy and more oxygen to do low-level activities compared to women with adequate magnesium levels. A multivitamin might provide the magnesium you need. Also reach for bran cereals, nuts, and fish, especially halibut, for good sources.

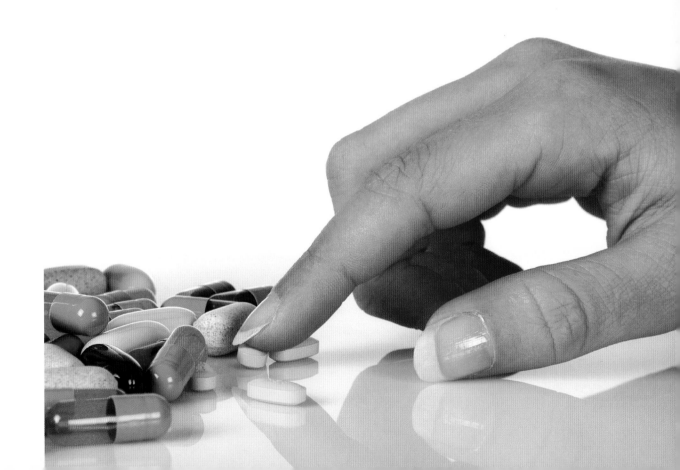

Poor Eating Habits **?**

In addition to the food and energy connections already mentioned, other habits cause energy levels to sag, including eating too much at once, eating the wrong kind of carbohydrates, drinking too much caffeine, and not getting enough fluids.

The Food Fix: Start each day by eating breakfast. After you fast all night, the body's blood sugar levels lower, and you simply must fuel up to gain some steam. Best breakfast choices include protein — yogurt, cottage cheese, low-fat milk or soymilk—with a complex carbohydrate such as a whole grain cereal or bagel. Skip the sticky cinnamon buns; the refined sugar they contain sends blood sugar levels soaring, only for them to plummet by midmorning.

If you tend to get sluggish after eating meals, reduce the amount of food you eat at one sitting. Spread out the food into smaller, minimeals. Some people function more efficiently with a consistent dose of calories throughout the day.

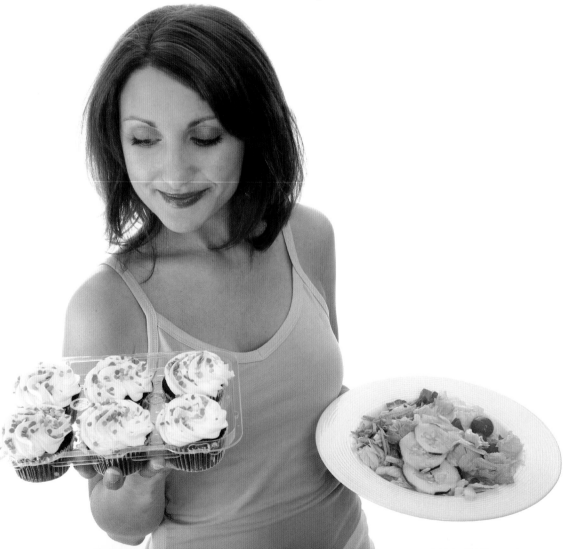

Photograph: www.istockphoto.com/ Sharon Dominick

Dehydration?

Caffeine, in small doses, increases your heart rate and provides a quick rush of energy needed by midday, but too much caffeine often has just the opposite effect. Drinking too much coffee or caffeinated soda leaves you feeling jittery and cranky.

The Food Fix: If you feel as if caffeine impairs a good night's sleep or leaves you wiped out at the end of the day, switch to decaffeinated products or reduce the amount of caffeine you drink.

Dehydration is often overlooked as a cause of fatigue. The Institute of Medicine's most recent fluid guidelines call for a person to drink about 11 cups per day from a variety of sources. Water, tea, coffee, juice, soda, and high-moisture fruits and vegetables all contribute to your daily hydration needs. Don't wait for thirst to guide you; fill up on fluids as a proactive measure. ❈

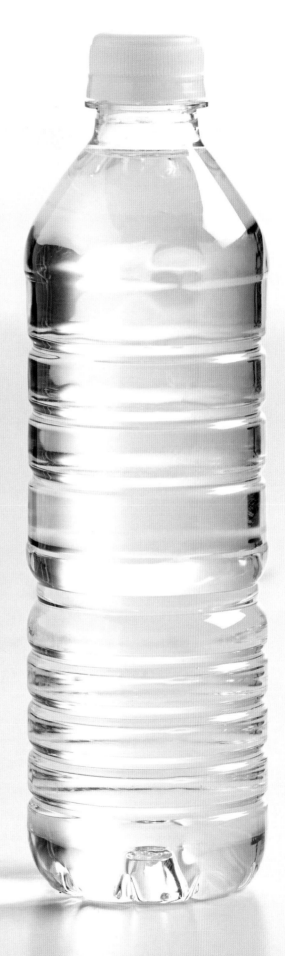

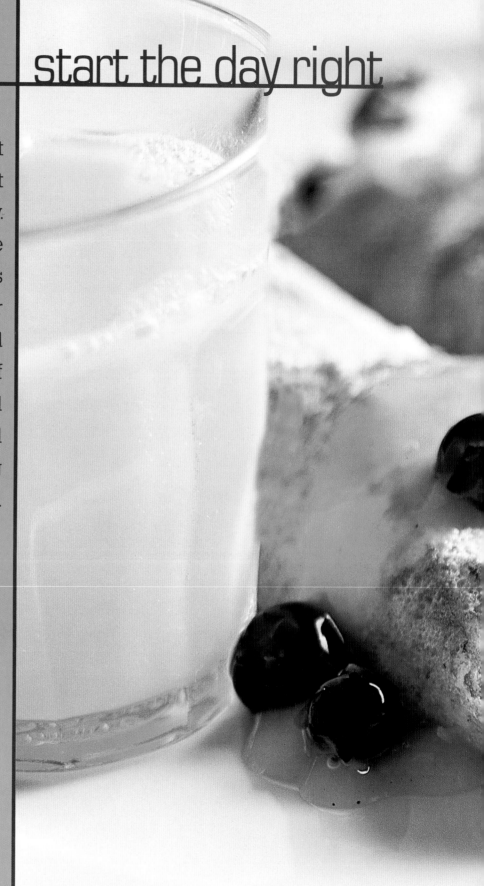

start the day right

A healthful breakfast offers the first step to a great day. Prepare any of the scrumptious dishes in this chapter for your family, and you'll send everyone off with the energy and nutrients needed to keep going all morning.

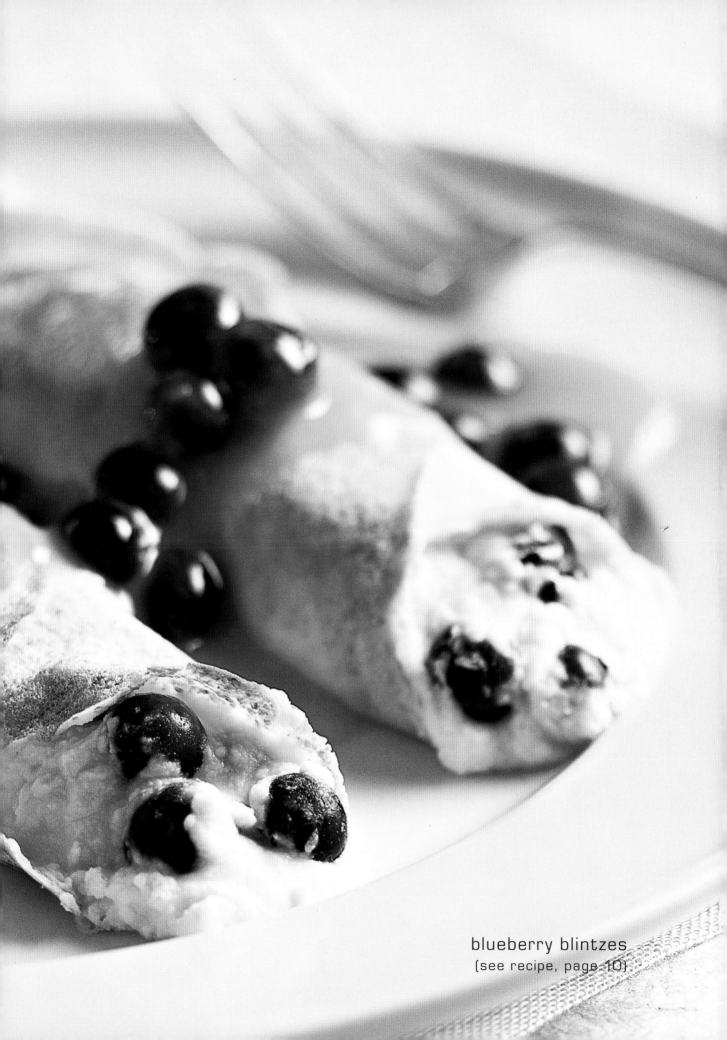

blueberry blintzes
(see recipe, page 10)

blueberry blintzes (see photo, pages 8-9)

The naturally sweet, juicy blueberries in this spectacular brunch dish provide antioxidants and calcium to keep your body healthy and strong.

Prep: 30 minutes
Bake: 15 minutes
Makes: 8 servings

  2   eggs
1⅓ cups fat-free milk
  ¾   cup whole wheat flour
  1   Tbsp. cooking oil
  ¼   tsp. salt
  1   15-oz. carton part-skim ricotta cheese
  2   cups blueberries
  ¼   cup packed brown sugar
1½ tsp. finely shredded orange peel
  1   cup orange juice
  1   Tbsp. cornstarch
  1   Tbsp. granulated sugar
  ¼   tsp. ground cardamom

1 Preheat oven to 400°F. For crepes, in a medium bowl combine eggs, milk, flour, oil, and salt; beat until well mixed. Heat a lightly greased 6-inch skillet over medium heat; remove from heat. Spoon in 2 tablespoons batter; lift and tilt skillet to spread batter. Return to heat; cook on one side only for 1 to 2 minutes or until brown. Invert over clean white paper towels; remove crepe. Repeat with the remaining batter, lightly greasing skillet occasionally.

2 For filling, in another medium bowl combine ricotta cheese, 1 cup of the blueberries, the brown sugar, and 1 teaspoon of the orange peel. Fill each crepe, browned side down, with a rounded tablespoon of the filling. Roll up crepe. Place blintzes in a 3-quart rectangular baking dish. Bake for 15 to 20 minutes or until heated through.

3 Meanwhile, for sauce, in a small saucepan stir together the remaining ½ teaspoon orange peel, the orange juice, cornstarch, granulated sugar, and cardamom. Cook and stir until thickened and bubbly. Cook and stir for 2 minutes more. Stir in the remaining 1 cup blueberries. Spoon sauce over blintzes.

PER SERVING: 229 cal., 8 g total fat (3 g sat. fat), 70 mg chol., 181 mg sodium, 31 g carbo., 2 g fiber, 11 g pro.

tofu-and-veggie breakfast burritos

These spicy burritos feature protein-rich tofu to boost your energy level. The mild-tasting soy food takes on the flavors of the foods with which it's paired.

Start to Finish: 35 minutes
Makes: 8 servings

2 tiny new potatoes, cut into ½-inch cubes
1 medium zucchini, cut into thin bite-size strips
1 medium red sweet pepper, thinly sliced
½ cup finely chopped onion
3 cloves garlic, minced
1 Tbsp. olive oil
1 12- to 16-oz. pkg. extra-firm tofu (fresh bean curd), cut into ½-inch cubes
½ cup water
3 Tbsp. tamari or reduced-sodium soy sauce
2 tsp. curry powder
1 vegetable or chicken bouillon cube
8 8- to 10-inch spinach flour tortillas

1 In a covered medium saucepan cook potato in a small amount of boiling, lightly salted water for 10 to 12 minutes or until tender; drain.

2 Meanwhile, for filling, in a large nonstick skillet cook zucchini, sweet pepper, onion, and garlic in hot oil over medium heat about 5 minutes or until vegetables are tender. Stir in potato, tofu, water, tamari, curry powder, and bouillon cube. Cook about 10 minutes more or until most of the liquid is evaporated, stirring occasionally.

3 Wrap tortillas in microwave-safe paper towels. Microwave on 100% power (high) for 30 to 60 seconds or until tortillas are warm.

4 To serve, spoon filling down center of each tortilla. Fold one end to partially cover filling; roll up from an adjacent side. Serve immediately.

PER SERVING: 291 cal., 6 g total fat (0 g sat. fat), 2 mg chol., 1,133 mg sodium, 47 g carbo., 2 g fiber, 12 g pro.

Note: If you need only four burritos for breakfast, cover and chill half of the filling for up to 2 days. To serve, transfer filling to a microwave-safe container; cover with waxed paper. Microwave on 100% power (high) for 2½ to 3½ minutes or until heated through, stirring once. Heat and fill tortillas as above.

three-grain flapjacks

For a tasty fiber boost, top these wholesome pancakes with fruit. If your favorite fresh fruit isn't in season, choose a frozen, canned, or bottled version.

Start to Finish: 30 minutes
Makes: 8 to 10 servings

1½ cups all-purpose flour
½ cup yellow cornmeal
2½ tsp. baking powder
½ tsp. salt
½ cup regular rolled oats
3 Tbsp. packed brown sugar
1 egg, beaten
1¾ cups light milk
¼ cup plain low-fat yogurt
3 Tbsp. cooking oil
½ cup dried blueberries or
  currants (optional)
Nonstick cooking spray
Pure maple syrup or reduced-
  calorie maple-flavor syrup
  (optional)

1 In a large bowl stir together flour, cornmeal, baking powder, and salt. In a blender or food processor combine oats and brown sugar. Cover and blend or process until oats are coarsely ground. Stir oat mixture into flour mixture. Make a well in the center of flour mixture.

2 In a medium bowl combine the egg, milk, yogurt, and oil. Add the egg mixture all at once to flour mixture. Stir just until moistened (batter should be lumpy and thin). Let stand for 10 minutes to thicken slightly, stirring once or twice. If desired, gently fold in blueberries.

3 Lightly coat a nonstick griddle or heavy skillet with cooking spray. Heat over medium heat.

4 For each pancake, pour about ¼ cup batter onto the hot griddle or skillet. Cook over medium heat for 1½ to 2 minutes or until pancakes have bubbly surfaces and edges are slightly dry. Turn pancakes; cook for 1½ to 2 minutes more or until golden brown. If desired, serve the pancakes with syrup.

PER SERVING: 233 cal., 8 g total fat (4 g sat. fat), 62 mg chol., 624 mg sodium, 68 g carbo., 4 g fiber, 14 g pro.

wheat germ and carrot muffins

Wake up to one of these great-tasting muffins. The wheat germ provides vitamin E, and the carrots are loaded with vitamin A.

Prep: 15 minutes
Bake: 20 minutes
Makes: 12 servings

Nonstick cooking spray
1 cup golden raisins or dried currants
2 cups all-purpose flour
⅓ cup toasted wheat germ
1½ tsp. baking powder
½ tsp. baking soda
½ tsp. salt
½ tsp. ground cinnamon
1 egg, beaten
1¼ cups buttermilk
½ cup packed brown sugar
¼ cup cooking oil
1 cup shredded carrot

1 Preheat oven to 400°F. Lightly coat twelve 2½-inch muffin cups with cooking spray. In a small bowl pour enough boiling water over raisins to cover them; set aside.

2 In a medium bowl combine the flour, wheat germ, baking powder, baking soda, salt, and cinnamon. Make a well in the center of flour mixture.

3 In a small bowl combine the egg, buttermilk, brown sugar, and oil. Add the egg mixture all at once to flour mixture. Stir just until moistened (batter should be lumpy). Drain raisins. Gently fold raisins and carrot into batter.

4 Spoon batter into the prepared muffin cups, filling each about three-fourths full. Bake about 20 minutes or until muffins are golden brown. Cool muffins in pan on a wire rack for 5 minutes. Remove from muffin cups. Serve warm.

PER SERVING: 226 cal., 6 g total fat (1 g sat. fat), 19 mg chol., 242 mg sodium, 39 g carbo., 2 g fiber, 5 g pro.

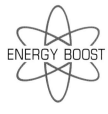

ENERGY BOOST

Soak your fatigue away. Take a hot bath. Warm water loosens tight muscles and relieves stress, leaving you with more energy. A hot soak erases a day's tensions and leaves you ready to face your evening with a little bit of pep. Plus the relaxing soak will help you sleep better.

Z's count!

by Michele Meyer

More than 100 million Americans of all ages each year fail to get good sleep. And we are suffering for it: from heart disease to depression to accelerated aging, the latest condition tied to sleeplessness. Yet bypassing bedtime is considered a virtue in corporate America, where high-powered executives crow about their five or fewer hours of sleep.

Though the average adult gets six hours and 58 minutes of Z's nightly, we actually need at least one hour more. Only 35 percent of adults get the desired eight hours of sleep.

Even the sleep we get isn't much to boast about: Two-thirds of us complain about having insomnia a few nights or more a week, reports a National Sleep Foundation poll. The complaints: waking up unrefreshed, struggling to fall asleep, rousing repeatedly during the night, or rising early and being unable to return to sleep. At least 42 percent of Americans are so sleep-deprived it harms their work and relationships.

While you were sleeping

You may seem completely out of it as you snooze, but deep within, your body works overtime. Your body alternates between 90-minute to two-hour cycles of deep, or slow-wave, sleep and REM, or rapid eye movement, sleep. During deep sleep, organs, bones, and tissues are repaired, while during REM, emotions and memories are processed. For the greatest benefit, you need at least eight hours of sleep with a high percentage of deep sleep in the first two hours and mostly REM sleep in the last two hours.

Throughout the night, your body tunes itself up, recharging your batteries, resetting your thermostat, and topping your fluids so you can operate at your peak. Your brain is the conductor, refurbishing your worn organs, burning calories, releasing hormones (including growth hormone, which builds muscle), and processing and storing the day's memories and lessons. All of your body's parts play their roles with the well-timed precision of a symphony orchestra. Instead of a major finale, this concert ends when your biological clock registers that you've paid off any sleep debt.

Interrupt the performance too early and you lose your rhythm. The results are crankiness, slowed

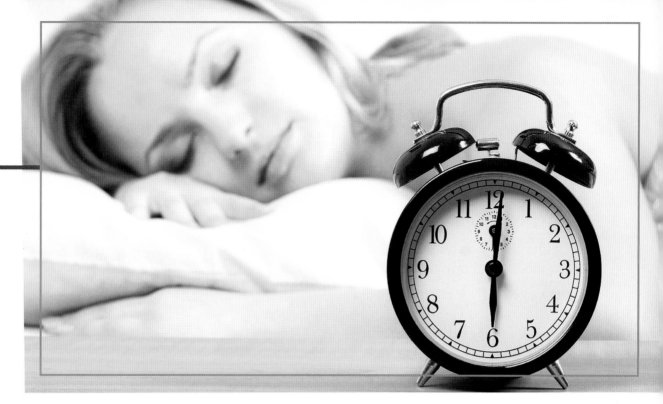

Photograph: www.istockphoto.com/ Alex Gumerov

reaction time, hampered creativity, inability to remember and make decisions, and most of all, drowsiness.

That's not all

Consider these tragedies:

• On his way from Springfield, Kentucky, to Crossville, Tennessee—a one-hour trip—James Rich put his twin-engine plane on autopilot. He woke up six hours later when his gasless plane crashed into the Gulf of Mexico. Though the U.S. Coast Guard rescued Rich, he lost his pilot's license and ruined the $70,000 plane.

• Robert Gaito, an Albany, New York, computer programmer who had been working overtime, thought he had dropped off his 5-month-old son at the babysitter on the way to work. Only after his wife called that evening when she got to the sitter did he check and find his son still in the car.

• Remember *The Exxon Valdez?* The oil tanker slammed into an Alaskan reef in 1989. About 11 million gallons of oil were dumped, requiring a $2 billion coastal cleanup—all due to a sleepy third mate at the wheel.

The price we pay

Sleep deprivation causes an estimated 100,000 accidents a year on the road, according to the National Transportation and Safety Board. Insomniacs are 3.5 to 4 times more likely to be in a car accident and 1.5 times more likely to be in a workplace accident.

Combining alcohol with sleeplessness can be lethal. Having one drink of alcohol on six hours of sleep affects your ability to drive the same as if you'd had six drinks on eight hours of sleep.

An inadequate amount of sleep can shorten your life in more ways than one. A University of Chicago study of 11 healthy men, ages 17 to 28, found that when their sleep was restricted

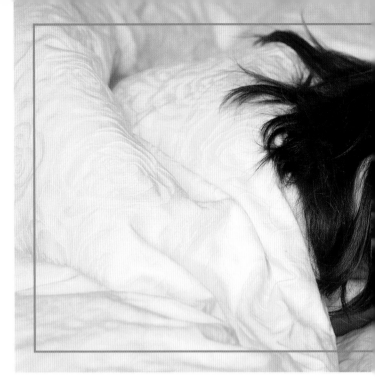

to four hours each night for six nights in a row, they aged rapidly. Their levels of hypertension, diabetes, and memory problems rose to levels usually associated with 60-year-olds. Fortunately, as reported in the United Kingdom medical journal *The Lancet,* the subjects were refreshed after a few nights of 12-hour slumbers.

Growing evidence shows that a lack of sleep makes us more vulnerable to infection, as well as high blood pressure, anxiety, weight gain, and stress. Insomniacs have a higher risk of developing depression. Other normal activities, such as eating, drinking, or having sex, take just a few minutes, but your sleep needs require an extended period of sleep every day.

Going without sleep can be your greatest error. Sleep loss will kill you on the highway, erode your productivity, and ruin you on the job. If you don't take sleep deprivation seriously, you'll pay the price. You might drop your dishes in the clothes dryer and not realize it until you turn the machine on and they shatter. You may fall asleep at a red light, waking only when the driver behind you honks. Or you could fall asleep during sex—not exactly conducive to romance. All have happened to sleep experts' patients.

The real danger is if we don't realize we're tired, we'll go about our

business as if we were capable. To return to full capacity, we need to repay our sleep deficit. Indeed, sleep debt is much like a financial one. Once you rob your dozing bank, you need to refill it with the same amount, ideally by oversleeping for several days.

How sleep needs change with age
The more your body is growing, the more slumber you need. Infants doze 16 or more hours a day; 3-year-olds only 12 hours. From puberty to age 20, a child needs nine hours and 15 minutes. Throughout adulthood, most of us need eight hours of sleep. But starting at age 40, our deep, restorative sleep begins to decrease. Shut-eye becomes disrupted due to medications, pain, and other health problems. Our internal clocks also send us to bed and wake us up earlier. Yet while sleep may be tougher to get, our sleep needs don't lessen.

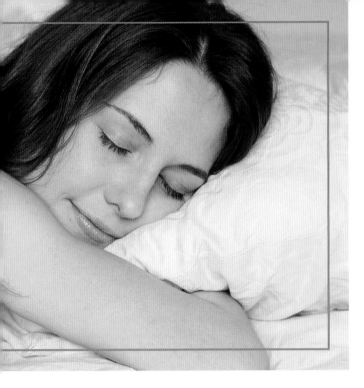

Get a better night's sleep

The best way to get maximum rest is to practice the following:
* Go to bed and wake up at the same time each day. Use bright light in the morning and dim bulbs in the evening to cue your internal clock.
* Refrain from acidic foods, such as orange juice, or spicy foods. These may induce heartburn that disrupts sleep. Eat your last meal at least three hours before bedtime.
* Exercise regularly. This deepens and extends sleep. Don't work out within three hours of going to bed because exercise raises your body temperature, which can make sleep more elusive.
* Review your medications with a doctor. Antihistamines, decongestants, blood pressure medicine, beta-blockers, and pain medications can disturb sleep.
* Establish a relaxing nighttime ritual, perhaps reading or listening to gentle music. Keep your bedroom secure and comfortable, darkened with shades or lined drapes. Try shutting out noise with earplugs, white noise, or rugs that absorb sound.
* Consider a mattress with individual pocketed coils to avoid being disturbed by your partner's movements. Choose a pillow, preferably down, that keeps your head, neck, and spinal cord in a straight line. Replace the pillow if it won't spring back when you fold it.
* From three to six hours before lights-out, cut off any stimulants, such as nicotine, coffee, soft drinks, and tea. Also, avoid alcohol after dinnertime. It may make you fall asleep quickly, but it causes light, fragmented dozing.
* If you don't fall asleep within 15 minutes, don't fret. Go to another room to read or listen to soothing music.

If you don't take sleep deprivation seriously, you will pay the price.

If you suffer insomnia for more than three weeks, keep a sleep diary for four to seven days to show your doctor. Record when you went to bed, fell asleep, woke up during the night, how you felt in the morning, and the timing of drinks and exercise. Your doctor may prescribe—usually for less than a month's duration—drugs such as newly developed Ambien and Sonata, both of which leave the body quickly so you're not groggy in the morning. ✳

go meatless

Nutrient-rich grains, beans, fruits, and vegetables make these meatless dishes not only good for you but also delicious and satisfying. Whether you want to cook meatless often or just now and again, you'll find these hearty, full-flavored entrées sure to please.

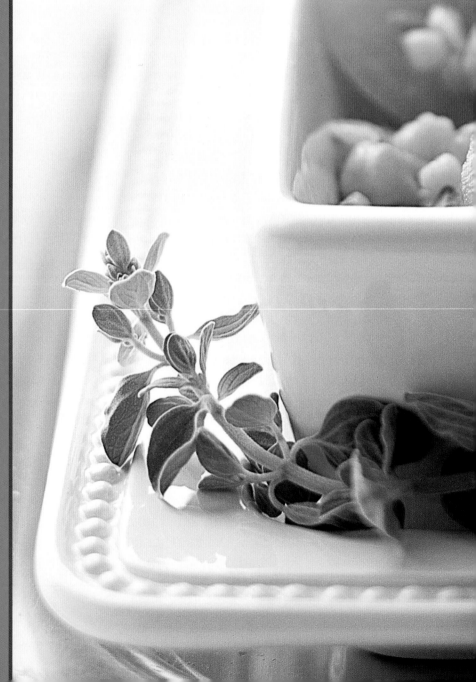

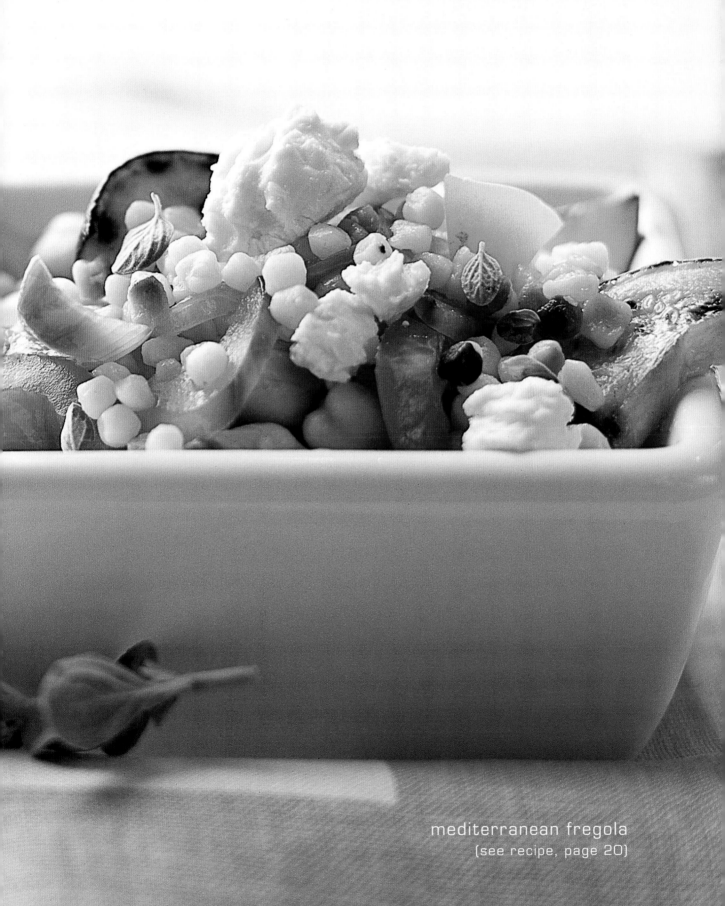

mediterranean fregola
(see recipe, page 20)

mediterranean fregola (see photo, pages 18–19)

Fregola is not a grain; it is a tiny pasta. Fregola and garbanzo beans pair up in this meatless dish to provide a complete source of protein.

Start to Finish: 25 minutes
Makes: 4 servings

6 cups water
1 Tbsp. instant chicken bouillon granules
1½ cups fregola (Italian couscous) or dried orzo pasta (rosamarina)
1 Tbsp. olive oil
1 medium red onion, halved lengthwise and thinly sliced
2 medium zucchini and/or yellow summer squash, halved lengthwise and sliced ¼ inch thick
¼ tsp. salt
¼ tsp. ground black pepper
1 Tbsp. small fresh oregano leaves or 1 tsp. dried oregano, crushed
1 clove garlic, minced
2 cups chopped roma tomato
1 15-oz. can garbanzo beans, rinsed and drained
½ cup crumbled feta cheese (2 oz.)

1 In a large saucepan bring water and bouillon granules to boiling. Add fregola. Cook according to package directions; drain. Transfer to a large bowl. Drizzle with 1 teaspoon of the oil; toss to coat. Cover and keep warm.

2 Meanwhile, in a large nonstick skillet heat the remaining 2 teaspoons oil over medium heat. Add the onion; cook for 2 minutes. Add zucchini, salt, and pepper. Cook for 3 to 4 minutes or just until zucchini is tender, stirring frequently. Stir in oregano and garlic; cook for 1 minute more. Stir in tomato and garbanzo beans; heat through.

3 Spoon the vegetable mixture over fregola; toss gently to coat. Divide among four bowls or dinner plates. Sprinkle with feta cheese. If desired, garnish with additional fresh oregano leaves.

PER SERVING: 430 cal., 10 g total fat (3 g sat. fat), 13 mg chol., 1,268 mg sodium, 72 g carbo., 5 g fiber, 17 g pro.

bean quesadillas with tomatillo salsa

This quick and tasty meal offers almost half of your daily fiber needs. Fat-free refried beans and reduced-fat cheese keep the fat and calories in check.

Prep: 15 minutes
Bake: 5 minutes
Makes: 6 servings

8 oz. fresh tomatillos, husked, stems removed, and cut into quarters (about 8)
1 small red onion, cut up
¼ cup fresh cilantro leaves
1 fresh jalapeño chile pepper, seeded and cut up
1 Tbsp. lime juice
¼ tsp. salt
Nonstick cooking spray
1 16-oz. can fat-free refried beans
½ tsp. ground cumin
½ tsp. chili powder
6 10-inch flour tortillas
1½ cups fresh corn kernels, cooked (about 3 medium ears), or 1½ cups frozen whole kernel corn, thawed
2 cups shredded reduced-fat cheddar cheese (8 oz.)

1 For salsa, in a food processor combine tomatillo, red onion, cilantro, jalapeño pepper, lime juice, and salt. Cover and process with several on-off turns until mixture reaches desired consistency.

2 Preheat oven to 350°F. Coat two large baking sheets with cooking spray. In a medium bowl stir together refried beans, cumin, and chili powder.

3 Place tortillas on a work surface. Spread half of each tortilla with the refried bean mixture. Top with the corn; sprinkle with 1½ cups of the cheese.

4 Lift the unspread side of each tortilla up and over the spread side; press lightly. Place tortillas on baking sheets; sprinkle tops with the remaining ½ cup cheese.

5 Bake about 5 minutes or until cheese is melted. Cut the quesadillas into wedges and serve with salsa.

PER SERVING: 380 cal., 11 g total fat (5 g sat. fat), 27 mg chol., 847 mg sodium, 48 g carbo., 7 g fiber, 19 g pro.

Note: Because chile peppers contain volatile oils that can burn your skin and eyes, avoid direct contact with them as much as possible. When working with chile peppers, wear plastic or rubber gloves. If your bare hands do touch the peppers, wash your hands and nails well with soap and warm water.

two-bean burritos

Hearty, high-protein beans provide an abundant source of compounds called saponins that are thought to control cholesterol and triglyceride levels.

Prep: 20 minutes
Cook: 10 minutes
Makes: 6 servings

- 6 10-inch spinach flour tortillas
- 1 15-oz. can black beans, rinsed and drained
- 1 8¾-oz. can whole kernel corn, rinsed and drained
- 1 medium mango, chopped (1 cup)
- ⅓ cup chopped red sweet pepper
- ¼ cup snipped fresh cilantro
- 2 Tbsp. lime juice
- 1 fresh jalapeño chile pepper, seeded and finely chopped (see note, page 21)
- ½ cup chopped onion
- 2 tsp. olive oil or cooking oil
- 1 16-oz. can vegetarian refried beans
- ½ cup salsa

1 Preheat oven to 350°F. Wrap the tortillas in foil. Bake about 10 minutes or until warm.

2 Meanwhile, in a medium bowl combine half of the black beans, the corn, mango, sweet pepper, cilantro, lime juice, and jalapeño pepper. Set aside.

3 In a large skillet cook onion in hot oil about 5 minutes or until onion is tender. Stir in the remaining black beans, the refried beans, and salsa; heat through.

4 Divide the refried bean mixture among the warm tortillas; roll up tortillas. Top each serving with corn mixture.

PER SERVING: 308 cal., 7 g total fat (1 g sat. fat), 0 mg chol., 871 mg sodium, 69 g carbo., 9 g fiber, 12 g pro.

vegetable-polenta lasagna

Polenta deliciously substitutes for noodles in this lasagna. For the most fiber, vitamins, and minerals, purchase water- or stone-ground cornmeal.

Prep: 25 minutes
Chill: 1 hour
Bake: 40 minutes
Makes: 8 servings

  4 cups cold water
1½ cups cornmeal
1¼ tsp. salt
  1 small onion, thinly sliced
  1 Tbsp. olive oil
  4 cups fresh mushrooms, halved
  ¼ tsp. freshly ground black pepper
  6 medium red and/or green sweet peppers, roasted and cut up, or two 12-oz. jars roasted red sweet peppers, drained and cut up
1¼ cups marinara sauce
  1 cup shredded mozzarella cheese (4 oz.)

1 For polenta, in a medium saucepan bring 2½ cups of the water to boiling. In a medium bowl combine the remaining 1½ cups water, the cornmeal, and 1 teaspoon of the salt. Slowly add cornmeal mixture to boiling water, stirring constantly. Cook and stir until mixture returns to boiling; reduce heat to low. Cook about 10 minutes or until mixture is very thick, stirring occasionally.

2 Pour the hot mixture into a 3-quart rectangular baking dish. Cool slightly. Cover and chill about 1 hour or until firm. (Or cover and chill for up to 24 hours.)

3 Preheat oven to 350°F. In a large nonstick skillet cook onion in hot oil over medium heat for 3 to 4 minutes or until tender. Add mushrooms, black pepper, and the remaining ¼ teaspoon salt. Cook and stir about 5 minutes or until mushrooms are tender. Remove from heat; stir in the roasted sweet pepper.

4 Spread the marinara sauce over chilled polenta. Top with the vegetable mixture and sprinkle with mozzarella cheese. Bake, covered, for 30 minutes. Uncover and bake for 10 to 15 minutes more or until edges are bubbly.

PER SERVING: 203 cal., 6 g total fat (2 g sat. fat), 8 mg chol., 597 mg sodium, 31 g carbo., 5 g fiber, 8 g pro.

the new power lunch

by Gary Thompson

Fitting a good workout into a busy schedule seems a challenge. If you get up early to exercise, you may find your body well rested but your mind still asleep. At the end of the day, your spirit may be willing but your flesh weak. Meet your body's schedule halfway: Exercise at lunch.

A noontime workout offers the perfect solution for busy people. Not only does it provide a break in the day, it also allows you to get stimulated for a full afternoon of work.

In response to employees' desire to work out at lunch, businesses often set up on-site fitness facilities and classes or offer reduced-price access to nearby health clubs. Such arrangements provide employers a happier, healthier workforce, while employees gain convenient and inexpensive access to professional equipment and instruction.

You don't need a fancy fitness center or health club to get the benefits of a lunchtime workout. Take a walk, run, ride a bike, or just take the stairs instead of an elevator to accumulate the 30 minutes of daily exercise recommended by most fitness experts.

The best exercise for you depends on your goals, according to the American Council on Exercise (ACE). If you want to lose weight, the ACE says to consider low- or no-impact aerobic routines, working up to 30 minutes per day. If you want to build muscle, use free weights, machines, or calisthenics to help tone and define your muscles. If you want improved flexibility, try yoga or a simple stretching routine that covers all major muscle groups. If you do an intense workout— running, fast walking, aerobics, weight lifting—you need to allow time for a shower.

The other main drawback to lunchtime exercise is you sacrifice a leisurely meal. Though exercising at noon means changing your eating habits, don't skimp on pre- or post-workout meals. Your body needs even more fuel to run in high gear when you exercise. You don't want to exercise on an empty stomach. If you eat breakfast at 7 a.m. and don't consume anything else before a noon workout, your body will be low on energy and your workout will suffer.

Though it's tempting to believe that eating less and exercising more

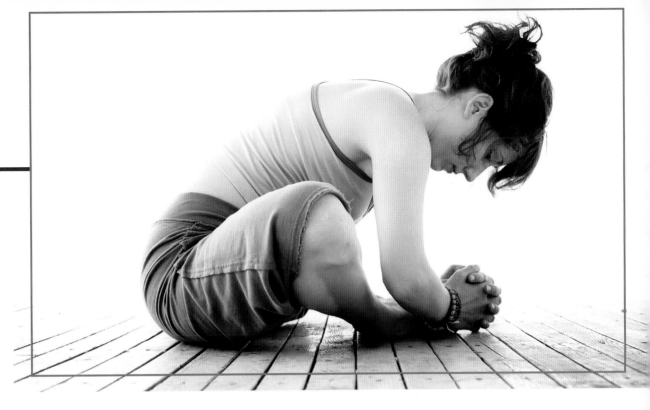

Photograph: www.istockphoto.com/ Valentin Casarsa

sheds pounds and burns fat faster, experts say the opposite is true. When deprived of calories, the body burns calories and fat more slowly as a survival technique. Keep your energy level up and your metabolism working at an optimum rate by eating small meals throughout the day.

Experts recommend you eat some carbohydrates—such as a piece of fruit or a bagel—about one hour before your workout. It's also important to drink plenty of fluids before, during, and after exercise. Popular sports drinks offer a good source of carbohydrates, but some newer varieties also contain a lot of sugar. Study nutritional labels to find a sports drink that contains 14 to 15 grams of carbohydrates per 8-ounce serving.

Your thirst may be up after your workout, but you probably won't be hungry. As body temperature rises with exercise, appetite decreases; however, an hour or two later, as the body cools, the appetite rebounds with a vengeance. Don't ignore your body's cry for fuel. If you try to hold out until dinner, you'll face a feeding frenzy when you get home. Don't head for the vending machines either. Break out the sandwich you packed for lunch or eat a nutritious minimeal. Good choices include peanut butter and fruit preserves on whole grain bread or a combination of a banana, a carrot, and 1 ounce of whole grain crackers.

Whichever way you choose to balance your food and exercise needs, a midday workout provides more than just physical benefits. People who work out at lunch seem happy and relaxed. A fitness break at lunch, experts say, serves as an effective stress-management technique. ✳

power meals

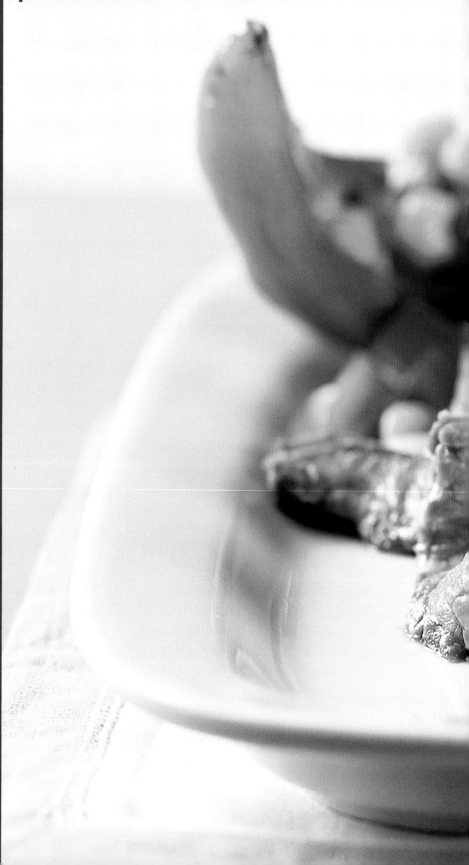

Building meals around hearty beef, pork, and lamb main dishes ensures your family develops the energy and vitality for an active lifestyle. These entrées—everything from steak and stir-fries to soups and salads to curries and kabobs—provide the zip you all need.

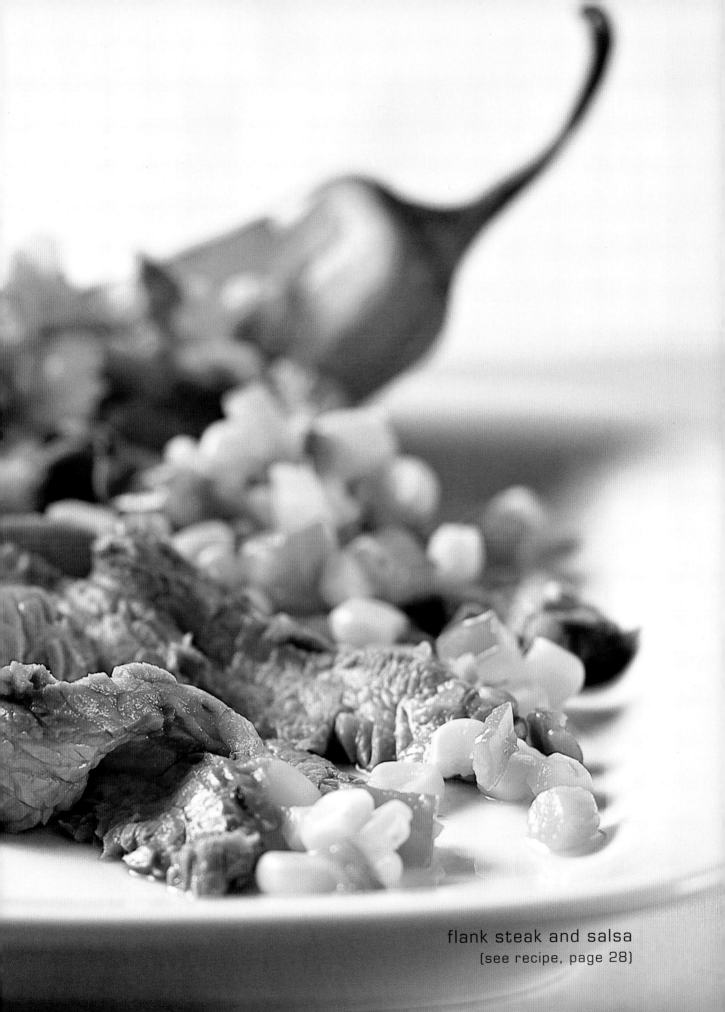

flank steak and salsa
(see recipe, page 28)

flank steak and salsa (see photo, pages 26–27)

With only 197 calories and 10 grams of fat, this Italian-seasoned steak provides a lot of protein and energy without sabotaging a healthful diet.

Prep: 15 minutes
Marinate: 6 hours
Broil: 15 minutes
Makes: 6 servings

- 1 8¾-oz. can whole kernel corn, drained
- ¾ cup salsa verde
- 1 medium tomato, chopped
- 1 1¼- to 1½-lb. beef flank steak
- ¾ cup Italian salad dressing
- 2 Tbsp. cracked black pepper
- 1 Tbsp. Worcestershire sauce
- 1 tsp. ground cumin

1 For salsa, in a medium bowl combine corn, salsa verde, and tomato. Cover and chill for 6 to 24 hours.

2 Meanwhile, trim fat from meat. Score both sides of meat in a diamond pattern by making shallow diagonal cuts at 1-inch intervals. Place meat in a resealable plastic bag set in a shallow dish.

3 For marinade, in a small bowl combine salad dressing, pepper, Worcestershire sauce, and cumin. Pour over meat; seal bag. Marinate in the refrigerator for 6 to 24 hours, turning bag occasionally. Drain meat, discarding marinade.

4 Preheat broiler. Place meat on the unheated rack of a broiler pan. Broil meat 3 to 4 inches from the heat until desired doneness, turning once. (Allow 15 to 18 minutes for medium doneness.)

5 To serve, thinly slice meat diagonally across the grain. Serve meat with salsa.

PER SERVING: 197 cal., 10 g total fat (0 g sat. fat), 44 mg chol., 313 mg sodium, 9 g carbo., 2 g fiber, 19 g pro.

stir-fried beef, broccoli, and tofu

Excellent served with brown rice or another cooked whole grain, this dish contains a healthy dose of fresh broccoli and protein-rich tofu.

Prep: 30 minutes
Marinate: 2 hours
Cook: 8 minutes
Makes: 4 servings

8   oz. boneless beef sirloin steak, cut ¾ inch thick
3   Tbsp. reduced-sodium soy sauce
3   Tbsp. rice wine
1   Tbsp. cornstarch
1   Tbsp. grated fresh ginger
2   tsp. sugar
2   cloves garlic, minced
8   oz. extra-firm tub-style tofu (fresh bean curd), drained and cut into ½-inch cubes
½   cup reduced-sodium chicken broth
2   Tbsp. cooking oil
4   cups broccoli florets
3   cups hot cooked brown rice

1 Trim fat from meat. Cut meat across the grain into thin bite-size strips. Place strips in a medium bowl.

2 For marinade, in a small bowl combine soy sauce, rice wine, 2 teaspoons of the cornstarch, the ginger, sugar, and garlic. Pour half of the marinade over meat. Add tofu to the remaining marinade. Gently stir both meat and tofu mixtures to coat with marinade. Cover and marinate in the refrigerator for 2 hours, stirring both mixtures occasionally.

3 Drain meat and tofu, reserving the marinades. For sauce, in a small bowl combine marinades, broth, and remaining 1 teaspoon cornstarch; set aside.

4 In a large nonstick skillet heat 1 tablespoon of the oil over medium-high heat. Add meat; cook and stir for 2 to 3 minutes or until meat is slightly pink in the center. Remove from skillet.

5 Add the remaining 1 tablespoon oil to skillet. Add broccoli; cook and stir for 2 minutes. Add tofu; cook and stir gently for 2 minutes. Return meat to skillet. Stir sauce; add to skillet. Cook and stir gently until mixture is bubbly. Cook for 1 minute more. Serve with brown rice.

PER SERVING: 426 cal., 14 g total fat (3 g sat. fat), 27 mg chol., 578 mg sodium, 45 g carbo., 5 g fiber, 26 g pro.

grilled pork and pepper skewers

Chile peppers add plenty of iron, zinc, vitamin C, and B vitamins to your diet, increasing your immunity to illness and improving your moods.

Prep: 20 minutes
Marinate: 4 hours
Grill: 12 minutes
Makes: 4 servings

- 12   oz. boneless pork top loin roast
- 2   medium red sweet peppers, cut into 1-inch pieces
- 1   medium red onion, cut into 1-inch pieces
- 1   6-oz. carton plain low-fat yogurt
- 3   green onions, thinly sliced
- 2   canned chipotle chile peppers in adobo sauce, finely chopped (see note, page 21)
- 2   Tbsp. snipped fresh parsley
- 1   Tbsp. grated fresh ginger
- 2   cloves garlic, minced
- 1   tsp. sugar
- 1   tsp. ground coriander
- ¼   tsp. salt
- ⅛   tsp. ground black pepper
- Hot cooked brown rice (optional)

1 Trim fat from meat. Cut meat into 1-inch pieces. Place meat, sweet pepper, and red onion in a medium bowl.

2 For marinade, in a small bowl stir together yogurt, green onion, chipotle pepper, parsley, ginger, garlic, sugar, coriander, salt, and black pepper. Pour over meat mixture, stirring to coat. Cover and marinate in the refrigerator for 4 to 6 hours, stirring occasionally.

3 When assembling the kabobs, wear plastic or rubber gloves to protect your hands from the oils in the chipotle pepper marinade. On eight 6- to 8-inch metal skewers alternately thread meat, sweet pepper, and red onion, leaving ¼ inch between pieces.

4 Grill kabobs on the rack of an uncovered grill directly over medium coals for 12 to 14 minutes or until meat is slightly pink in the center, turning once halfway through grilling. If desired, serve the kabobs with brown rice.

PER SERVING: 184 cal., 3 g total fat (1 g sat. fat), 53 mg chol., 298 mg sodium, 14 g carbo., 2 g fiber, 24 g pro.

harvest pork soup

Root vegetables complement tender pork in this herbed soup. They also help increase your immunity, boost energy, and fight cancer and heart disease.

Start to Finish: 30 minutes
Makes: 6 servings

- 10 oz. boneless pork top loin chops, cut ¾ inch thick
- 1 Tbsp. cooking oil
- 5 cups beef or chicken broth
- 2 cups cubed, peeled sweet potato
- 1 cup sliced carrot
- 1 cup chopped onion
- 1 cup chopped, peeled turnip
- ½ cup sliced celery
- ½ cup quick-cooking pearl barley
- 1 Tbsp. snipped fresh oregano or ½ tsp. dried oregano, crushed
- 1 Tbsp. snipped fresh sage or ½ tsp. ground sage
- ¼ tsp. ground black pepper

1 Trim fat from meat. Cut the meat into ¾-inch pieces. In a 4-quart Dutch oven cook the meat in hot oil over medium heat for 4 to 5 minutes or until meat is brown. Drain off any fat.

2 Add broth, sweet potato, carrot, onion, turnip, celery, barley, dried oregano (if using), ground sage (if using), and pepper.

3 Bring to boiling; reduce heat. Simmer, covered, for 12 to 15 minutes or until vegetables are tender. If using, stir in fresh oregano and sage.

PER SERVING: 215 cal., 5 g total fat (1 g sat. fat), 30 mg chol., 717 mg sodium, 26 g carbo., 4 g fiber, 16 g pro.

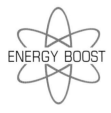

ENERGY BOOST

Starting a meal with soup helps you consume fewer calories. According to a study at Baylor College of Medicine in Houston, hot soup partially fills your stomach so you eat less later in the meal.

pork with black beans and succotash

Tex-Mex dishes often get their spicy taste from salsa. Tomato salsas contain the antioxidant lycopene, which may reduce the risk of prostate cancer.

Start to Finish: 20 minutes
Makes: 4 servings

8 to 10½ oz. low-fat bulk pork sausage
½ cup chopped onion
½ cup chopped red sweet pepper
1 10-oz. pkg. frozen succotash or 1 cup frozen whole kernel corn plus 1 cup frozen lima beans
¼ cup water
1 15-oz. can black beans, rinsed and drained
½ cup salsa
2 Tbsp. snipped fresh cilantro
8 6-inch corn tortillas
1 small avocado, seeded, peeled, sliced, and halved
Light dairy sour cream (optional)

1 In a large nonstick skillet cook sausage, onion, and sweet pepper about 5 minutes or until meat is brown. Drain off fat. Stir in succotash and water.

2 Bring to boiling; reduce heat. Simmer, covered, about 15 minutes or until lima beans in succotash are tender. Stir in black beans and salsa. Heat through. Remove from heat. Stir in cilantro.

3 Meanwhile, preheat oven to 350°F. Wrap tortillas in foil. Bake about 10 minutes or until tortillas are warm. Serve sausage mixture with tortillas, avocado, and, if desired, sour cream.

PER SERVING: 392 cal., 5 g total fat (1 g sat. fat), 33 mg chol., 717 mg sodium, 66 g carbo., 10 g fiber, 24 g pro.

beat the afternoon slump

Ugh. It's midafternoon. The late-day doldrums known as the slump have hit. Cure the sluggish feeling with one or more of these four slump-busting tips whether you're at home or in the office.

SWAP OUT COFFEE

Your first thought might be to reach for some java, but it won't help pep you up for long. Caffeine only temporarily blocks the signals to your brain that let you know you're tired.

At the office: Sip decaffeinated herbal tea, water with lemon, or fruit juice. All are reinvigorating.

At home: Whip up a fruit smoothie. The mix of complex carbohydrates and simple sugars in the fruit will energize you.

GET ON THE LAUGH TRACK

Chortles raise your endorphin levels and make you feel better almost instantly.

At the office: Do something lighthearted like singing a silly song to yourself. Or take a break with a coworker who always makes you laugh.

At home: Talk back to your radio or TV, or don't just talk, yell. Soon you'll crack yourself up and feel better.

EAT SMALL

Because in midafternoon you haven't eaten for a few hours, the blood sugar that keeps your brain alert is low.

At the office: Rev up with a small snack such as a 6-ounce cup of yogurt and half of an energy bar. Avoid sweets from the vending machines. They'll just make you crash again in an hour.

At home: Try a bowl of whole grain cereal with low-fat milk or peanut butter on whole wheat toast.

TAKE A HIKE

Even a few minutes of walking helps snap you out of the doldrums.

At the office: Instead of sending an e-mail, walk to a coworker's office to talk. To really get a boost, walk the stairs a few times.

At home: Get outside for some fresh air and sunlight instead of staying inside under artificial light. Take a cruise around the block or plan outdoor chores, such as gardening, for midafternoon.

the lighter side

A terrific strategy for giving everyone in the family an energy boost is to serve lighter, more healthful meals. These taste-tempting chicken, turkey, fish, and seafood recipes offer just the inspiration you need.

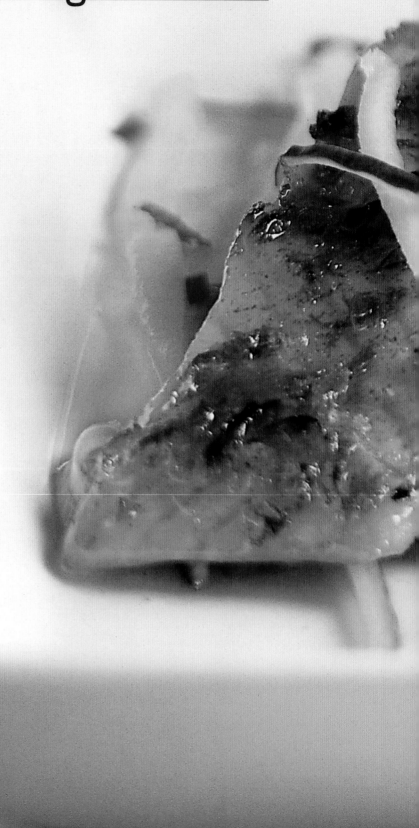

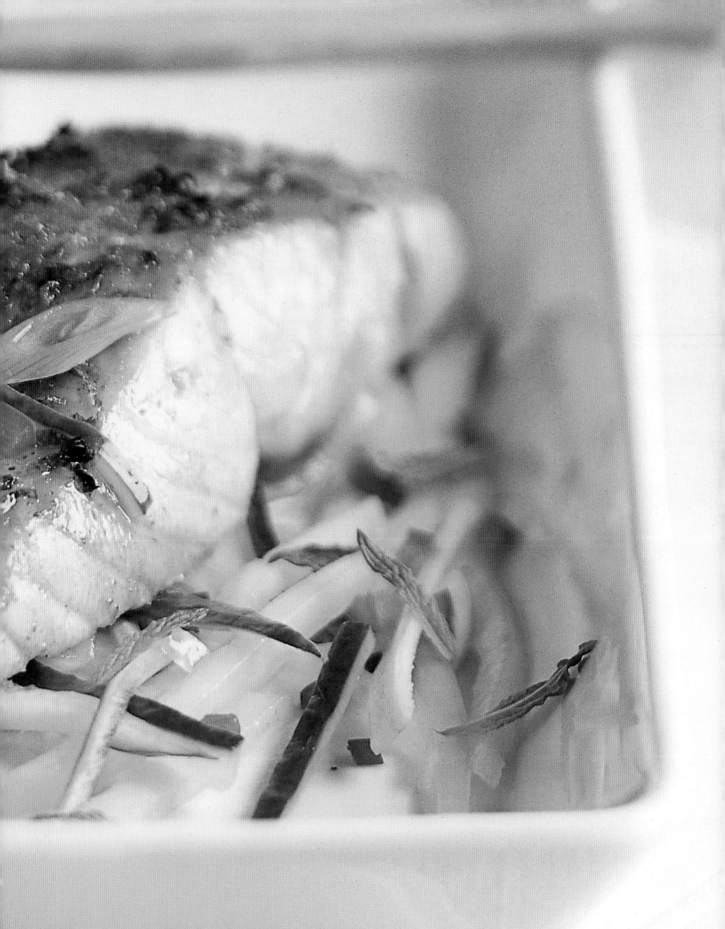

salmon with mango salsa
(see recipe, page 36)

salmon and mango salsa (see photo, pages 34–35)

This recipe packs a dietary punch. The omega-3-rich salmon boosts energy levels and lifts moods. Mango contains a lot of vitamins A, C, and E.

Prep: 15 minutes
Marinate: 4 hours
Grill: 14 minutes
Makes: 4 servings

- 4 6- to 8-oz. fresh or frozen salmon fillets (with skin), 1 inch thick
- 2 Tbsp. sugar
- 1½ tsp. finely shredded lime peel
- ¾ tsp. salt
- ¼ tsp. cayenne pepper
- 1 large ripe mango, seeded, peeled, and cut into thin bite-size strips
- ½ of a medium cucumber, seeded and cut into thin bite-size strips
- 2 green onions, sliced
- 3 Tbsp. lime juice
- 1 Tbsp. snipped fresh cilantro or 2 tsp. snipped fresh mint
- 1 small fresh jalapeño chile pepper, seeded and chopped (see note, page 21)
- 1 clove garlic, minced

1 Thaw fish, if frozen. Rinse fish; pat dry with paper towels. Place fish, skin sides down, in a shallow dish.

2 For rub, in a small bowl stir together sugar, lime peel, ½ teaspoon of the salt, and the cayenne pepper. Sprinkle rub evenly over fish; rub in with your fingers. Cover and marinate in the refrigerator for 4 to 24 hours.

3 Meanwhile, for salsa, in a medium bowl combine mango, cucumber, green onion, lime juice, cilantro, jalapeño pepper, garlic, and the remaining ¼ teaspoon salt. Cover and chill until ready to serve.

4 In a grill with a cover arrange medium-hot coals around a drip pan. Test for medium heat above the pan.

5 Place fish, skin sides down, on the greased grill rack over drip pan, tucking under any thin edges. Cover and grill for 14 to 18 minutes or until fish flakes easily with a fork. If desired, remove skin from fish. Serve the fish with salsa.

PER SERVING: 352 cal., 15 g total fat (3 g sat. fat), 105 mg chol., 520 mg sodium, 18 g carbo., 2 g fiber, 37 g pro.

grilled turkey with pepper sauce

Loaded with vitamin C, red and yellow sweet peppers add natural sweetness to the savory sauce atop these grilled turkey steaks.

Prep: 20 minutes
Grill: 25 minutes
Makes: 4 servings

2 Tbsp. olive oil or cooking oil
2 medium red or yellow sweet peppers, chopped
½ cup finely chopped onion
¾ cup chicken broth
¼ tsp. salt
¼ tsp. ground black pepper
2 cloves garlic, minced
2 turkey breast tenderloins (about 1 lb. total)
3 cups hot cooked mafalda pasta or fettuccine
2 Tbsp. finely shredded fresh basil

1 For sauce, in a large skillet heat 1 tablespoon of the oil over medium heat. Add sweet pepper and onion. Cook about 10 minutes or until vegetables are very tender, stirring occasionally. Transfer vegetables to a food processor or blender; add broth, salt, and black pepper. Cover and process or blend until mixture is smooth. Return to skillet; set aside.

2 In a small bowl combine the remaining 1 tablespoon oil and the garlic. Brush the garlic mixture over turkey.

3 In a grill with a cover arrange medium-hot coals around a drip pan. Test for medium heat above the pan. Place turkey on the grill rack over the drip pan. Cover and grill for 25 to 30 minutes or until turkey is tender and no longer pink.

4 Cut the turkey into slices. Reheat the sauce. Serve the turkey and sauce over pasta. Sprinkle with basil. If desired, garnish with additional fresh basil.

PER SERVING: 380 cal., 9 g total fat (2 g sat. fat), 68 mg chol., 348 mg sodium, 38 g carbo., 3 g fiber, 34 g pro.

chicken in shiitake mushroom sauce

Carrots and tiny pearl onions provide the body enhanced immunity, anticancer benefits, heart protection, and healthier skin.

Prep: 20 minutes
Cook: 40 minutes
Makes: 4 to 6 servings

3 lb. meaty chicken pieces (breast halves, thighs, and drumsticks)

Salt

Ground black pepper

2 Tbsp. olive oil

8 oz. pearl onions

4 medium carrots, cut into 1-inch pieces

¼ cup dry vermouth

1 14-oz. can chicken broth

3 Tbsp. snipped fresh parsley

1 Tbsp. snipped fresh thyme

1 Tbsp. snipped fresh rosemary

8 oz. fresh shiitake mushrooms, halved

1 Skin chicken. Sprinkle chicken with salt and pepper. In a 12-inch skillet heat oil over medium heat. Add chicken. Cook about 10 minutes or until chicken is golden brown, turning to brown evenly. Remove chicken.

2 Add pearl onions and carrot to skillet. Cook about 5 minutes or until onions are golden brown, stirring occasionally. Add vermouth, scraping up any crusty browned bits from bottom of skillet. Return chicken to skillet. Pour broth over chicken; sprinkle with parsley, thyme, and rosemary.

3 Bring to boiling; reduce heat. Simmer, covered, about 40 minutes or until chicken is tender and no longer pink (170°F for breasts; 180°F for thighs and drumsticks), adding mushrooms the last 10 minutes of cooking. If desired, garnish with additional fresh rosemary.

PER SERVING: 446 cal., 20 g total fat (4 g sat. fat), 138 mg chol., 624 mg sodium, 14 g carbo., 4 g fiber, 50 g pro.

kale, lentil, and chicken soup

This flavorful home-style soup packs nutrients that help aid immunity, lift moods, strengthen bones, improve the skin, and increase energy.

Prep: 25 minutes
Cook: 30 minutes
Makes: 6 servings

1 Tbsp. olive oil
1 cup chopped onion
1 cup coarsely chopped carrot
2 cloves garlic, minced
6 cups reduced-sodium chicken broth
1 Tbsp. snipped fresh basil or 1 tsp. dried basil, crushed
4 cups coarsely chopped kale (about 8 oz.)
$\frac{1}{2}$ tsp. salt
$\frac{1}{8}$ tsp. ground black pepper
1$\frac{1}{2}$ cups cubed cooked chicken
1 medium tomato, seeded and chopped
$\frac{1}{2}$ cup red lentils, rinsed and drained

1 In a large saucepan heat oil over medium-low heat. Add onion, carrot, and garlic. Cook, covered, for 5 to 7 minutes or until vegetables are nearly tender, stirring occasionally.

2 Add broth and, if using, dried basil to vegetable mixture. Bring to boiling; reduce heat. Simmer, covered, for 10 minutes. Stir in kale, salt, and pepper. Return to boiling; reduce heat. Simmer, covered, for 10 minutes.

3 Stir in chicken, tomato, lentils, and, if using, fresh basil. Simmer, covered, for 5 to 10 minutes more or until kale and lentils are tender.

PER SERVING: 199 cal., 5 g total fat (1 g sat. fat), 31 mg chol., 871 mg sodium, 20 g carbo., 7 g fiber, 20 g pro.

life in the slow lane

by Gary Thompson

Many of us have turned life into a race, speeding along in a frantic attempt to get from one place to another as quickly as possible.

Not that races are bad. Completing a race is a tremendous physical and mental accomplishment, but you don't see much while you're running. What's more, to people watching the race, it appears the runners aren't having much fun. The runners' facial expressions—grim, determined, and revealing thirst, pain, and fatigue—express how badly the competitors wish the race was over. Is that how we look to disinterested bystanders as we rush around each day?

Yes, say people from other cultures. North Americans' frantic lifestyles frighten them. Though work serves as the main culprit, even at home, at play, or on vacation, North Americans live life at a high speed. We've gotten into the habit of cramming more in, whether it's more work or more pleasure.

The urge to cram as much into life as possible is hard to resist. Modern communication and transportation, along with our own expectations, push us to try to pack more and more into every day. Our expectations result in overscheduled hyperactivity and families so busy with scheduled events that they don't spend meaningful time together.

How do you know you're living too fast? Symptoms can be both physical and emotional. Usually a person feels a sense of vague discontent or a little nagging feeling that something's not quite right. It also may seem as if you're playing a role and only going through the motions. Just like a car possesses warning lights, the body sends certain physical signals—tense muscles, shallow breathing, rapid heartbeat, high blood pressure—to let you know when you're hitting the red zone. Ignoring these warnings can lead to bodily damage and breakdown.

In terms of dollars and cents, the highest cost of our breakneck pace occurs in the workplace. As employees, we rush to get more done, which results in more mistakes and the need to redo tasks. All of this decreases our productivity.

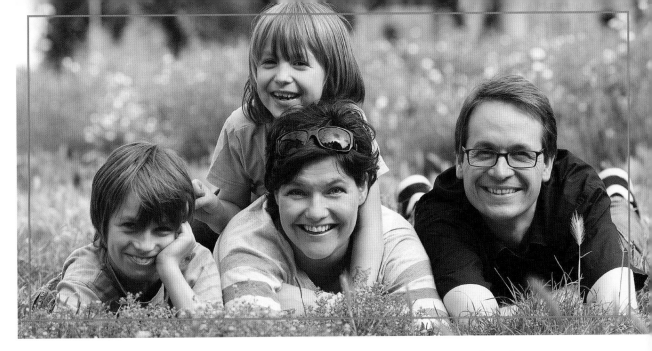

Photograph: www.istockphoto.com/ Wouter van Caspel

More costly in human terms are effects of hectic lifestyles on the home front. Couples spend less time alone, parents spend less time with children, and families don't do activities together. Gone are the days when families frequently enjoyed leisurely dinners, long drives, church services, birthday celebrations, and visits with relatives. Those little, regular rituals are the glue that holds together home and family life.

When your life gets overscheduled, it's not enough to simply practice deep breathing and tell yourself to relax. Truly slowing down combines a change in your external circumstances and the way you react to them. It means cutting the clutter from your schedule to make better use of your time:

Say no. When you need more time at home and more peace when you're there, politely but consistently say no to new work obligations or volunteer requests.

Tithe your time, donating only a percentage to a worthwhile cause as you would money to a church or charity. Be conscious of giving some time every week or month to something outside yourself.

Put feelings first. Listening to a child takes priority over balancing a checkbook. A romp with your dog is more important than waxing the floor. Everyday, repetitive chores can wait. Time spent with children or pets may not come again.

Prioritize. Make a list of tasks for each day and label each item with a letter. A priority item to be done today gets an *A*. *B* is for important items to be done soon. *C* indicates necessary items that should be done sometime. Get through the *A* items each day; then the *B* things become *A* projects, and the *C* items either rise or disappear.

Schedule fun. Don't downplay the importance of fun. Schedule time each week for sheer pleasure. Opt for activities that you enjoy that usually get crowded out of your schedule. No matter how much you try to simplify your life, you may not feel satisfied. It depends on your mind-set. If you don't enjoy the activities that fill your time, life can appear frantic even when it's not. Conversely, a seemingly stressful situation can be invigorating, even fun, if you live in the moment and enjoy new challenges.

Living in the present serves as the key to slowing down and enjoying life more. To live in the present, you need to see life as a series of moments—one right after another—and become fully engaged in each one, whether it's a conversation, work, a meal, or a game. Focus on

to move away from living in the moment as we get older. We need to recapture a childlike approach to life while still being responsible adults. "Living in the moment" doesn't mean a person lives an unstructured life, breaks commitments, misses appointments, or abandons schedules. Rather, it means you see each day as a series of satisfying experiences and let each event soak in.

"Slowing down" often means listening to your heart instead of your head. Whenever you look back on a day and find even one

Living in the present serves as the key to slowing down and enjoying life. You need to become so focused on an activity that you don't realize time is passing.

the here and now; don't analyze every move, fret about the next item on your schedule, or worry about tomorrow, next week, or next year.

When you live in the moment, you lose track of time, your senses become heightened, your thinking clears, your body feels good, and you come away from an experience emotionally satisfied.

Easier said than done? Perhaps. But once upon a time, everyone approached life that way. Children naturally live in the moment, losing themselves in play and finding joy in the simplest of activities. We all were children once, but we all tend

warm memory, you paid adequate attention to your heart. If following your heart leads you to take a detour in life, stay on the back roads, or stop to help someone along the way, the experience probably will be worth the time it took.

It may be difficult to find a warm memory every day, but if such moments seem rare in your life, perhaps you need to slow down. The trip called life doesn't last forever. Every moment you savor provides another souvenir to put on your mental mantel. Even if you know your destination, you can discover joy in the mundane parts of the journey. ✺

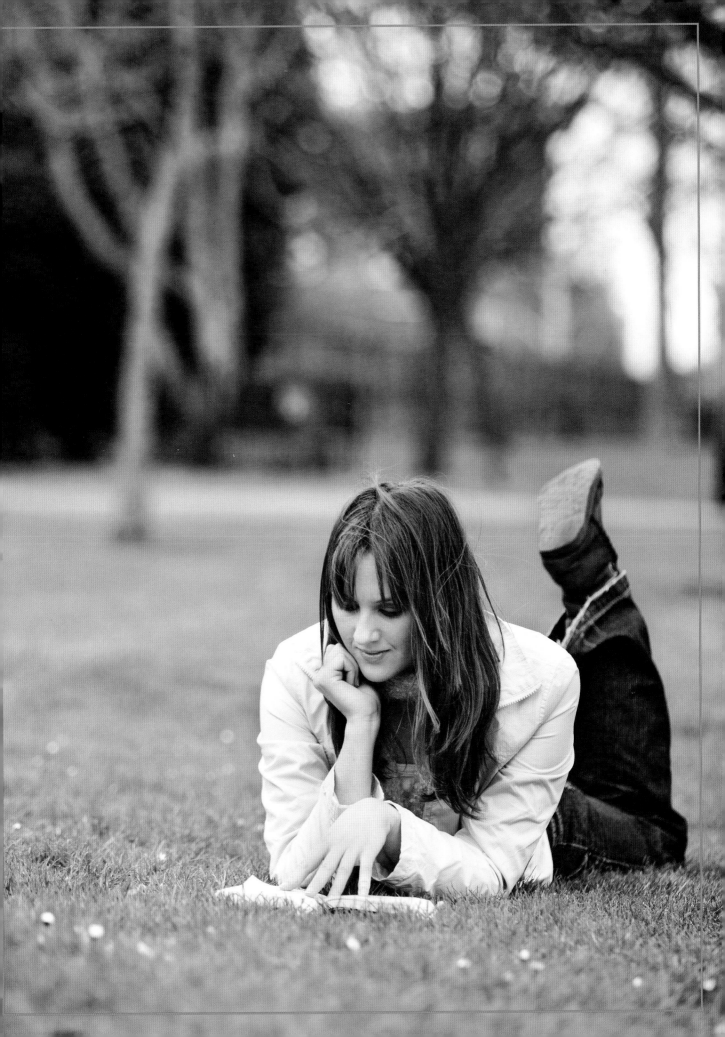

healthy sides

While healthy, energy-boosting meals start with nutritious main dishes, the recipes you select to fill out your menus are just as important. This collection of appealing serve-alongs completes good-for-you meals.

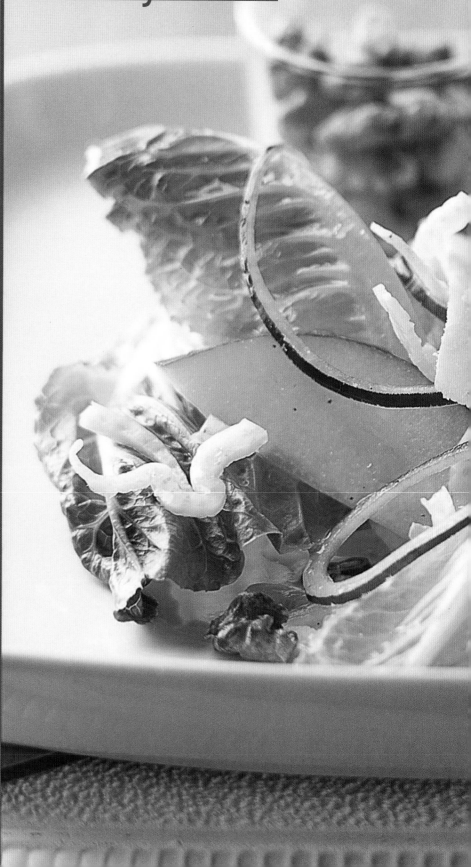

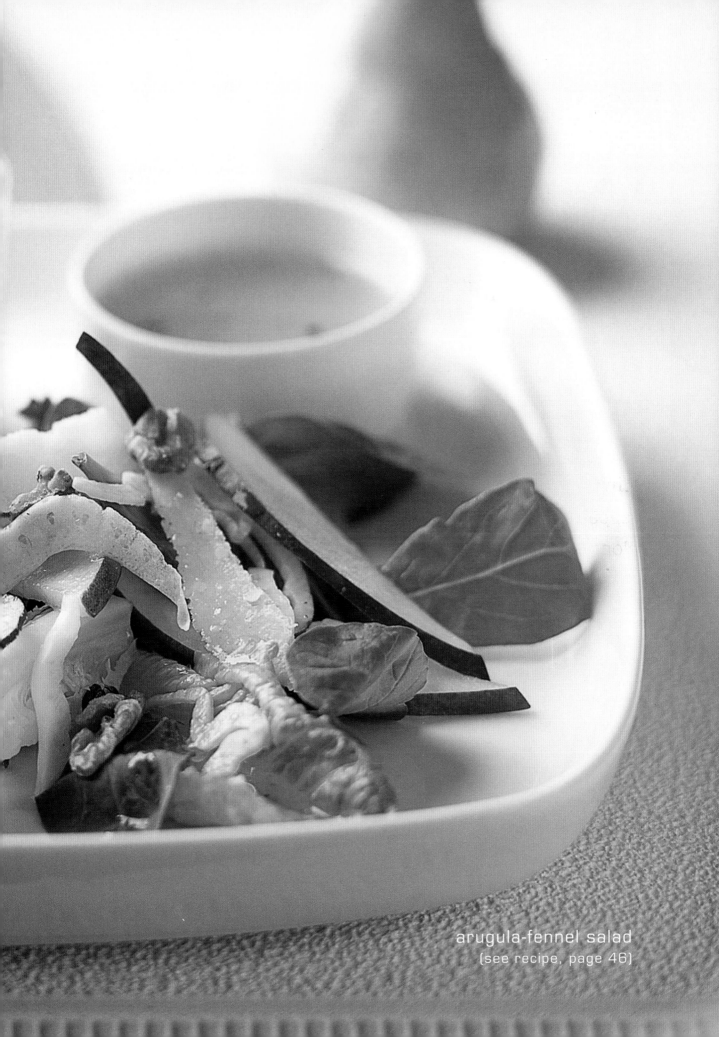

arugula-fennel salad
(see recipe, page 46)

arugula-fennel salad [see photo, pages 44–45]

Sweet, crisp pears loaded with soluble fiber and tossed with potassium- and calcium-rich fennel pack this salad with great taste and good nutrition.

Start to Finish: 25 minutes
Makes: 4 servings

2/3 cup pear nectar
3 Tbsp. seasoned rice vinegar
1 Tbsp. olive oil
1/2 tsp. coarsely ground black pepper
1 fennel bulb
2 cups arugula leaves
2 cups romaine lettuce leaves
2 small ripe pears, cored and thinly sliced
1/2 of a small red onion, thinly sliced and separated into rings
1/4 cup broken walnuts, toasted
1 oz. Parmesan cheese

1 For vinaigrette, in a bowl whisk together pear nectar, rice vinegar, oil, and pepper.

2 Cut off and discard upper stalks of fennel, reserving some feathery leaves for garnish (if desired). Remove wilted tough outer layer of stalks and cut a thin slice from base of bulb. Cut the fennel bulb in half lengthwise. Cut halves crosswise into thin slices, removing core (if desired).

3 In a medium bowl toss together sliced fennel, arugula, and romaine lettuce. Pour about half of the vinaigrette over fennel mixture; toss to coat. Arrange the fennel mixture on four salad plates. Top each serving with pear, red onion, and walnuts.

4 Use a vegetable peeler to thinly shave Parmesan cheese. Top the salads with shaved cheese and, if desired, garnish with fennel leaves. Drizzle with the remaining vinaigrette.

PER SERVING: 217 cal., 11 g total fat (2 g sat. fat), 6 mg chol., 282 mg sodium, 28 g carbo., 5 g fiber, 6 g pro.

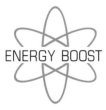

ENERGY BOOST

Take heart if you love nuts. Although long valued for their protein, vitamins, and minerals, nuts possess hidden talents as well. Nuts reduce the risk of heart disease. They're rich in fat, but mostly unsaturated fats—the same kinds that give olive oil its good name. Nuts also are great sources of fiber. Enjoy nuts in small amounts of unsalted varieties in salads, rice dishes, cereals, cakes, and muffins.